FIT LIFE, HAPPY LIFE

One Man's Journey

Kyle Juracek, PhD

ISBN 979-8-89112-421-9 (Paperback)
ISBN 979-8-89112-422-6 (Digital)

Covenant Books
11661 Hwy 707
Murrells Inlet, SC 29576
www.covenantbooks.com

ACKNOWLEDGMENT

The idea for this book was actually proposed by a friend of mine at the gym. We were discussing my lifetime of fitness and discipline one day when he said, "You should write a book." Without his suggestion, I don't think this book would have happened. Thanks, Dave!

CHAPTER 1

Introduction

What are the ingredients for a happy life? Financial stability, a career you enjoy, a nice home and car, a family, a loving and supportive spouse, good friends, and, most importantly, good health. Some people are blessed with all of these and more. Many are not. Whatever your situation is, I believe that adopting a healthy and active lifestyle, if you're physically able, will only improve your quality of life. If you're already living a healthy and active lifestyle, keep up the good work and keep enjoying the benefits!

In this book, you'll learn about my journey through life and some of the challenges I faced along the way. Through all of life's challenges, I have lived a healthy and active lifestyle and always managed to get my workouts in. I believe that has helped me maintain a positive attitude. Fundamentally, life is better with a positive attitude and worse with a negative attitude. I am fortunate because a positive attitude has always been a natural part of my personality. I've always had it, and I'm very grateful that I do.

My dedication to a healthy and active lifestyle has been essential to maintaining my physical and mental health and has only reinforced that positive attitude. If you're motivated, flexible, and creative at times, you will probably find that living a healthy and active lifestyle will be possible regardless of what life throws at you. You can do this, and you'll be glad that you did!

I hope you find my book to be interesting and informative. But, most of all, I hope it inspires you (at least a little) to live a healthy and active life that, ultimately, is a happier life too!

CHAPTER 2

The Teen Years

I was born in Lincoln and grew up in Omaha, Nebraska, in the 1960s and 1970s. Like a lot of boys growing up in Nebraska, I discovered Cornhusker football at an early age and became a huge fan. Since there were no pro teams to compete with, it was the main attraction. It was fun and easy to follow the Huskers back then as they were, and would be, really good for many years under Coach Tom Osborne.

In junior high school, I lived and died with the Huskers. If they won, it was going to be a good week. If they lost? Well, I didn't want to talk about it. At the time, I struggled to understand why they couldn't just win every game.

Naturally, it became my dream to one day play for the Huskers. How cool would that be? But, it was destined to be only a dream and a short-lived one at that. In my one and only season of playing organized football, in the ninth grade, I quickly discovered that I didn't have the hitter mentality that you have to have to be successful—that was strike one. I was big enough, athletic enough, and even really fast, but I didn't like to hit, and I didn't like getting hit. On top of that, I also discovered that I wasn't particularly competitive either—strike two. Finally, as I found out then and in future years, I tend to be a bit injury-prone—strike three. So playing for the Huskers was out.

I also dabbled in other sports—a few years of Little League baseball, a year on the sophomore basketball team in high school, three years throwing the shot put and discus in high school, although I couldn't use the spin technique for discus because my hands were too small. So the shot put became my favorite. I also liked throwing the shot, I think, because I was just competing with myself. But, maybe also because I could do it without injuring myself (or maybe I was just lucky!).

Anyway, my time as a competitive athlete ended in high school. I did briefly try the javelin in college, but it hurt my shoulder. It was during those high school years, though, that my interest in personal health and fitness emerged. At the age of seventeen, I made a promise to myself that I would always stay in shape. Okay, I admit that my personal health wasn't the only motivation. I also wanted to look good with the hope that it might help me get a girlfriend. Anyway, I'm happy to say that today, at age sixty-two, I've kept that promise. I'll tell you later about how I was able to stay motivated all those years.

During my senior year in high school, I joined my first gym. I'll never forget it. The gym was called Champion Charlie's Muscle Palace, and the owner was Charlie Brown. Honest, I'm not making that up. I started going to the gym every day after school to work out. One of my motivations was to get stronger for my senior season of shot and discus.

That would be the spring of 1979. I did improve my shot by three feet. My personal best that season was forty-six feet, three and three-fourth inches. I still remember. I was six feet two and weighed about 190 pounds. I never made my goal of fifty feet. But I did have one moment that I was proud of. On the day of that forty-six-foot throw, I defeated a rival from another high school who was six feet six and weighed about 250 pounds. That rival would go on to earn a football scholarship to Nebraska. He eventually became an all-American offensive lineman for the Huskers.

That first experience at a gym was memorable. I saw some really big guys throwing around a lot of weight. It was intimidating to a seventeen-year-old kid who had never lifted a weight before. But it was also motivating to see what might be possible with hard work. I remember one guy in particular that I admired because he had what were, in my eyes, shockingly big arms. Of course, at the time, I wanted to have big arms, too. Funny how your perspective can change dramatically as you age. Today, when I see someone with shockingly big arms, it strikes me as freakish, and I have no desire to possess such arms (and haven't for decades).

Here's some good advice: weight lifting can be dangerous; if you don't know what you're doing, ask someone who does. Sooner or later, if you use too much weight and (or) don't practice proper technique, it's probably only a matter of time before you suffer an injury. So be smart about it, ask for a spot if you need it, and don't forget to be observant of what's going on around you. In a gym with lots of equipment and moving parts, it can be surprisingly easy to get scraped, bruised, cut, or trip on something. One day in high school, I managed to have a twenty-five-pound plate drop edgewise on my toes. The pain was so intense that I couldn't even feel it at first. Then it came in throbbing waves. To this day, I still have a bone chip on my big toe from that day—a delightful souvenir from my early workout days.

Remember this: It's never too soon to start living a healthy and active lifestyle.

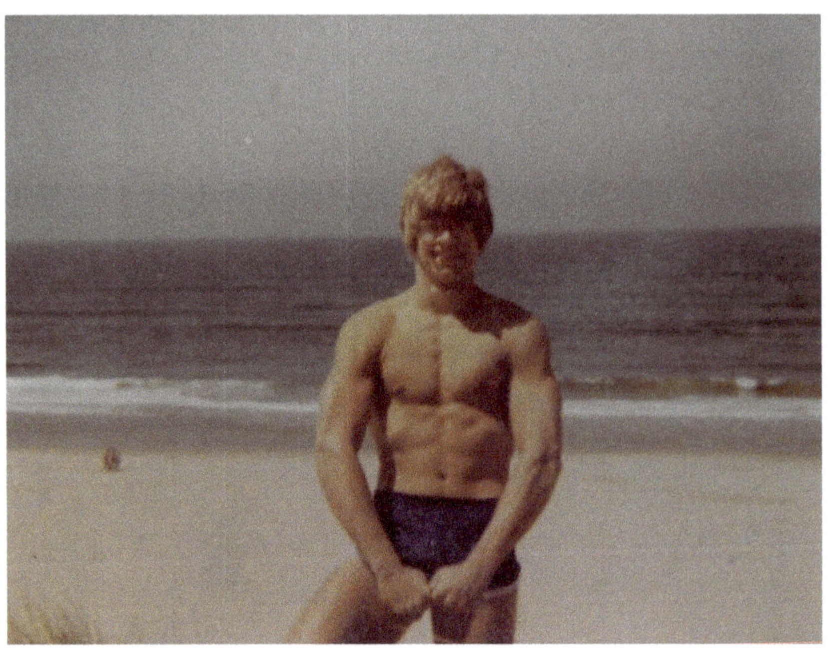

1979: Me at age eighteen

CHAPTER 3

The Twenties

My twenties unfolded in the 1980s: College; grad school; lots of good music, my favorite decade of music, actually; and, of course, lots of working out. As an undergrad, my priorities were, perhaps, a bit out of whack. Each semester, I would try to schedule my classes around my favorite workout time. For me, that was late morning, so I could go straight to lunch after. I hadn't yet figured out for sure what I wanted to do with my life, but I did know that staying in shape was important to me. For the health benefits and, yes, still to maybe impress girls. In an uncertain period of my life, I could always count on my workout to be part of each day. There was something reassuring about that, at least for me.

In my early twenties, I was very interested in getting bigger and stronger. I guess my motivation at the time was just simply to see how big and strong I could actually get. Steroids were everywhere in the 1980s, but that wasn't for me. I was never tempted. I was going to train naturally or not at all. I was very health conscious, and I wasn't about to do anything to jeopardize my health. So the answer for me was to train hard and train consistently. Eventually, I got my weight up to the 200- to 205-range. During this time, I set my personal records with a 320-pound bench and a 475-pound squat; pretty good. I briefly considered competitive powerlifting but quickly decided against it for two reasons. One, I figured I wouldn't be able to compete against the roid users. Two, I didn't want to hurt myself. I had already experienced some shoulder problems from heavy benching (and dips), and the deadlift kind of scared me.

I also briefly, very briefly, attempted to train for an amateur bodybuilding competition, but I didn't even last a week. It was the dieting that killed me; it sucked. The attempt ended while I was at a drive-in movie with a friend. While waiting for the first movie, I was thinking about how much the dieting sucked, and that was it. I went to the concession stand and got a corn dog. Damn, it was good.

It was a fun time, though—talking about favorite bodybuilders at the gym (Frank Zane was one of my favorites), getting pumped to "Eye of the Tiger," and reading muscle mags for the latest training tips. In 1981, I even went to the Mr. Universe contest in Columbus, Ohio, with one of my gym friends. I still have the T-shirt! Speaking of attire, I also had a nice collection of tank tops from different gyms.

Every once in a while, as an added bonus, you get to see a celebrity at the gym. One day, I walked into Champion Charlie's, and there was Jesse "The Body" Ventura hanging out and talking to everyone. In the 1980s, he was one of the best-known professional wrestlers. I assumed he must have been in town for some wrestling event, and yes, he was huge. I was never really a fan of professional wrestling, but it was still cool to see him. A few years later, at a Gold's Gym in California, I saw Chuck Norris, the TV and action film star—also cool.

Lifting impressive weights was a whole thing. You had to have the right gear and the right routine. Standard apparel for serious squatting included lifting shoes, a double-thickness leather belt, and knee wraps. And, if you were really serious, a tight-fitting, full-body lifting suit. But that wasn't all. To prepare for a really big lift, you also had to properly psych up. This could include pacing, chalking up, some slapping or pushing with your spotter friends, some yelling, and perhaps the use of some colorful language (i.e., swearing). Whatever it takes!

In the summer of 1986, a friend and I decided we wanted to do something athletic to impress ourselves before I left for graduate school, and he started law school. Inspired by Greg LeMond's win in the Tour de France that year (Note: He was the first rider outside of Europe to win the race), we decided that a big bike ride was going to be our impressive feat. So with little advance training, we hopped on our ten-speeds and rode fifty miles from Omaha to Lincoln on a narrow highway with no paved shoulder and lots of traffic—really stupid idea. We could have been killed or at least seriously injured. Somehow, we survived it unscathed. But to this day, I still wonder what the hell we were thinking.

In my late twenties, some things changed. My motivation to get big and strong faded for several reasons. For one, I kept hurting my shoulders. Those injuries forced me to give up two of my favorite exercises—bench press and dips. Fortunately, there are a number of other exercises available to work the chest and triceps, so I managed. Second, I came to realize that I didn't have the genetics to sculpt that perfect physique that I had worked so hard trying to achieve. In particular, my chest refused to grow. On the other hand, I had large, defined calves, and I didn't even train them—go figure. So for those two reasons, my motivation shifted away from bigger and stronger toward maintenance and health.

But there was also a third factor that came into play during my late twenties: those were my grad school years. As I progressed through grad school and approached the start of my professional career, the possibility occurred to me that having large muscles might compromise my image of being a competent professional. I didn't want to be perceived as a musclehead in a suit. Whether or not that was a valid concern is debatable. Regardless, in my mind, it was something to be aware of, not that I was ever freakishly large; I wasn't. Genetics would not permit that.

The story of my twenties would not be complete unless I told you about "garlic man." He was a middle-aged man who, apparently, believed very strongly in the health benefits of garlic. To that end, he ate it daily, as evidenced by the pronounced aura of stench that surrounded him when he entered the gym. I remember the dismay I felt every time I saw him coming. Talk about overcoming challenges to live a healthy and active lifestyle. Persevering through a workout in the presence of garlic man was no small feat—it took true dedication. Then, surprisingly, one day, he arrived at the gym without the stench. A joyous moment to behold! One way or another, he must have become aware of his foul stench and that it was very much not appreciated by fellow gym patrons, or maybe he was just tired of eating garlic. Either way, I was grateful!

The late twenties was an eventful time in my life: I met my wife, started my career, and took up permanent residence in Lawrence, Kansas, where I still live today.

Remember this: A healthy and active lifestyle will mean different things to different people. Discover what works for you and stick with it.

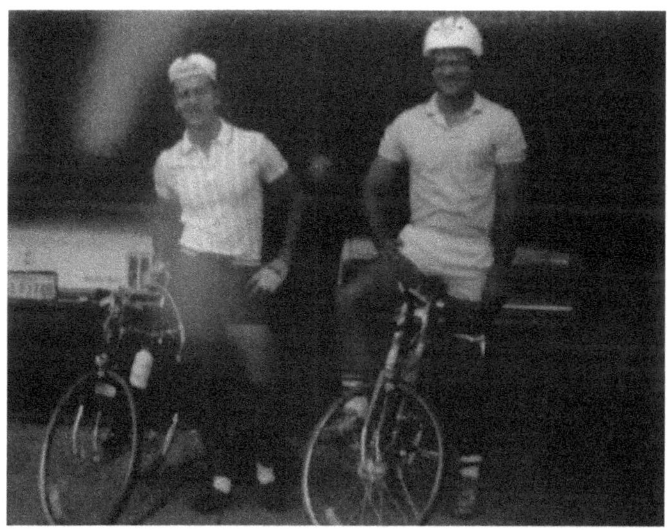

1986: My friend and I before embarking on our fifty-mile bike ride from Omaha to Lincoln. I was twenty-five at the time.

CHAPTER 4

The Thirties

"The best way to get in shape is to never get out of shape." I came up with that motto myself. And that's how I've lived my life.

In my thirties, life got busier, a lot busier. My wife and I were now both into our full-time careers, which occasionally involved some out-of-town travel, especially for me. And then our son was born in 1994, and we got a whole new appreciation for the importance of being patient and flexible. My family is in Nebraska, and her family is in California. So when our son was sick, the burden of care was totally on us.

At times, balancing career and family responsibilities was challenging, to say the least, and maximum flexibility was required. I remember one day in the summer of 1996 when our son was sick. Neither my wife nor I could take the full day off. I had to be out on a lake collecting samples while the weather was good and my crew was available. She had a can't-miss meeting that afternoon. So we came up with a plan. She stayed home with him that morning while I headed out to the lake. Early that afternoon, I got off the boat and drove forty-five minutes to meet her at an office building in Kansas City. After handing off our son to me, she attended her meeting. Afterward, I handed him back to her, drove back to the lake, got back on the boat, and continued sampling with the crew—quite the day.

Of course, the challenges of a busy life also impacted my workouts. I'm a planner, and I like to have a set daily schedule if possible. Now, I was finding that wasn't always going to be possible, and I had to learn to be okay with that. The important thing is not when you work out but that you work out. Over the years, I worked out at 5 a.m., 8 p.m., and everywhere in between. Sometimes work or travel would make it impossible to work out on a given day. When that happened, being the planner that I am, I would do a double workout the day before or after. I don't miss workouts! If it's truly a priority, you'll find the time, and I always did.

Traveling, work or personal, presented extra challenges. Beyond possible time constraints, sometimes access to equipment was a problem. Typically, the hotel would have an exercise room, but the quality varied widely. Some were surprisingly good and were equipped with free weights, benches, and an assortment of weight machines and cardio options. Others might only have a stationary bike and a treadmill. So you had to get creative with what you had. Occasionally, I had to get by with no equipment at all. If nothing else, I could always do push-ups, planks, and perhaps a power walk or jog. One time, I found a playground at a nearby school and did some pull-ups on the jungle gym. Something is always better than nothing!

It was during my thirties that I really, finally, appreciated the importance of cardio for total fitness and started making it a regular part of my weekly workout routine. In the past, I pretty much just lifted weights. I also did some activities with cardio benefits (for example, basketball, tennis, and bike riding), but not consistently. One year, I think it was 1992, I decided to see how many miles I could put on my ten-speed bike in a year. I had several different rural routes that I biked. In all, I biked 1,315 miles that year. For some people, that would be no big deal. But, for me, I was pretty proud of that accomplishment.

I don't know where it comes from, but I have always been very disciplined when it comes to my workouts. For me, workouts are not optional. It doesn't matter if I don't feel like working out that day. I do it anyway. Typically, once I get started, I'll get into it. Getting started is the key. And once the workout is finished, I'm always glad that I did it. The only time I ever miss a workout is when I'm really sick, which, thankfully, doesn't happen very often. I wish I could explain how to become disciplined when it comes to working out, but I can't. Maybe there's a good self-help book out there somewhere.

I do have a few suggestions for people struggling with discipline: try a training partner. Knowing that someone is counting on you to show up can be very motivating. I had a training partner from time to time over the years and enjoyed it. For me, it wasn't about needing an extra nudge to get to the gym. The big benefit for me was that we pushed each other during the workouts, so we both ended up getting better workouts as a result. The key is finding the right partner. Other suggestions I would offer include keeping a training journal, goal setting, and a reward system. I treat myself to ice cream every Friday. I love ice cream! It's my reward for a successful week of completing all my workouts and eating reasonably healthy. So I tell myself that I have to earn that ice cream.

As I got older, I got more serious about my diet. You realize that eating whatever you want whenever you want may not be the best idea, no matter how much you work out. I've always tried to keep it simple. I've never considered myself super strict when it comes to my diet, but others might disagree. I just try to eat reasonably healthy. Typically, I avoid fast food and anything deep-fried. I limit myself to red meat once a week. Mostly, I'll eat white meat and fish. I'm always trying to eat more vegetables and feel like I can always do better than I do. I'm a foodie, so I love good food. I also have a sweet tooth and love chocolate and, of course, ice cream. Thank goodness I'm pretty disciplined, or I'd really be in trouble!

For both the mental and physical benefits, it's important to stay active, and, of course, exercise is great for stress relief! Most people know these things. But, sadly, most people also don't do anything about it. Getting older doesn't, by definition, mean that you have to put on unwanted weight and develop health problems. For most people, it's a choice. Why not make a healthy choice?

Remember this: If your health is a priority (and it should be), you'll find the time.

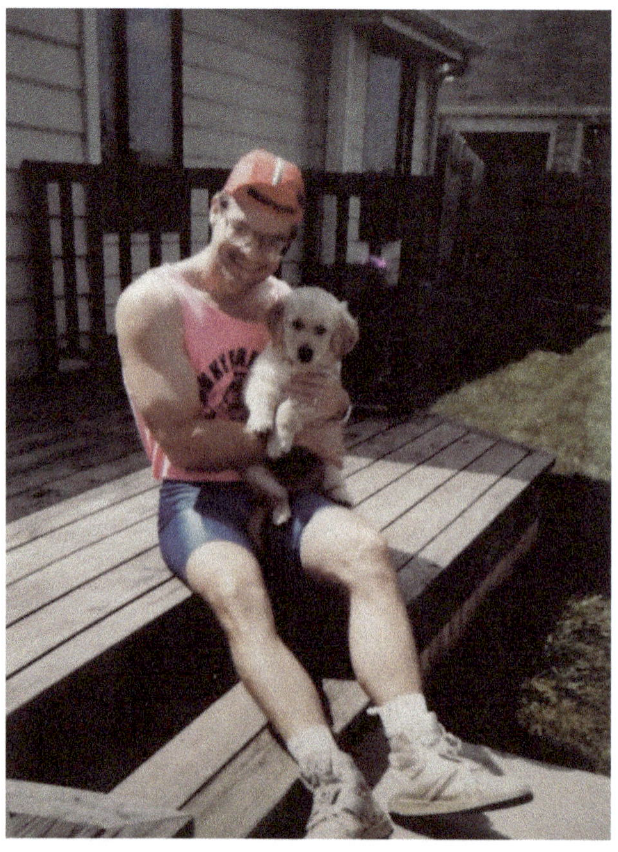

1992: Me at age thirty-one with my golden retriever Reggie, who was just a puppy at the time

CHAPTER 5

The Forties

If there's one thing I've learned from working out all these years, it is that you have to be smart about it. The older we get, the finer the line gets between pushing yourself for a good workout and hurting yourself. You have to learn to listen to your body. If something doesn't feel right, back off, don't push it. Good options include skipping that body part that day, using less weight, or perhaps trying different exercises that don't cause discomfort. And make sure you give yourself ample recovery time. I always wait at least three to four days before working on the same body part again. The older you get, the more important recovery becomes. Also, every three months, I take a week completely off from weightlifting to give myself a break, mentally and physically. I still do lots of cardio during those off weeks, though.

Another important consideration is the number of reps per set. Back when I was a young man, I would work my way up to heavy doubles and singles in exercises like the bench press and squat. I was always trying to set a new

PR (i.e., a personal record). And I kept hurting my shoulders as a result. So no more heavy doubles or singles. Now, for every exercise, I usually do six to twelve reps per set. Ideally, after one or two warm-up sets, every set is to failure (within that six- to twelve-rep target range). I choose weights that keep me in that target range.

Getting good exercise on vacation can sometimes be particularly challenging. One time, while on a family vacation in Estes Park, Colorado (elevation 7,500 feet), I scared the hell out of myself just trying to get a good cardio workout. We had brought our bikes on the trip. One day, I went for a ride. Most of the route was relatively flat. Then, I came upon a switchback (it was pretty steep and about a block long), and I brilliantly decided that I would do some climbs to get a really good cardio workout. Guess how many climbs I did: one. When I got to the top, my heart was pounding, and I was breathing so hard that my lungs were actually burning. I was scared to death that I was going to have a heart attack right then and there. I didn't, thank goodness, and after a few minutes of deep breathing, I recovered. I underappreciated the altitude effect that day, and I'll never make that mistake again—I hope.

It may sound strange, but after all these years of working out, it sometimes seems like my muscles are bored. It's gotten harder to get a good pump. Maybe that's just a part of aging. I've tried everything. I never do the same workout twice in a row. The number of sets and reps per set is fairly consistent, but I'll always do different exercises, or at least change the order of the exercises, every workout to try to keep the muscles guessing and hopefully get a better workout as a result. I used to think that I only had a good workout if I was sore the next day. But I now know that soreness is not a requirement to know whether or not you had a good workout.

One of the perks of joining a gym is the friends you make. Over the years, I made friends at several different gyms. I've found that having those friendships helped motivate me to go to the gym. Once at the gym, there's something to be said about being surrounded by other people who are working out. It's motivational. Enjoy the socialization, but try not to let it interfere with your workout. During my workouts, I always try to keep the socialization to a minute or less between sets so as not to lose my pump. That is, unless you're lifting really heavy weights, then more recovery time between sets is called for.

Personally, I enjoy messing with people at the gym and having them mess with me. It makes for some funny exchanges that leave everyone laughing; that's a good thing. Here's a sample of some of the things I've said: "You call that a set?" "You're using actual weights today? Impressive." And if I'm feeling particularly feisty: "Hey, if you aren't going to hit it with the proper intensity, then get the hell out." When someone I know is about to start using a piece of equipment, I've been known to say: "I was using that. I'm not now, but I was using it." And, finally, my profound and insightful philosophy on weight lifting: "It's not about how much weight you use, and it's not about proper technique. It's about making the right noises at the right time." I find that occasionally, being a smartass enhances my enjoyment of the gym experience. But only as long as the people on the receiving end know that you're kidding.

At this point, in my forties, I had been working out consistently for about thirty years. So what motivates me? The two most important considerations that have kept me motivated through the years are personal health and self-respect. Everywhere you look, you see unhealthy people. People who are overweight, some dangerously so, and people who have multiple health problems. Many health problems are caused, or made worse, by poor choices that include bad diet, lack of exercise, and a sedentary lifestyle. I have refused to become one of those people. Come to think of it, when I was sixteen, a twenty-five-year-old neighbor (who possessed an impressive belly) bet me $5 that I would have a gut by age twenty-five. I lost track of that neighbor over the years, but he still owes me that $5.

And then there's the self-respect. For me personally, self-respect has been one of the guiding lights for how I live my life. I strive to be a man that possesses the qualities I respect. Those qualities include honesty, integrity, discipline, modesty, and kindness. Additionally, my self-respect requires that I do everything I can to keep myself healthy and fit. I can't be out of shape. I can't.

Remember this: Motivations to be healthy and active will vary from person to person. Find what motivates you and focus on it.

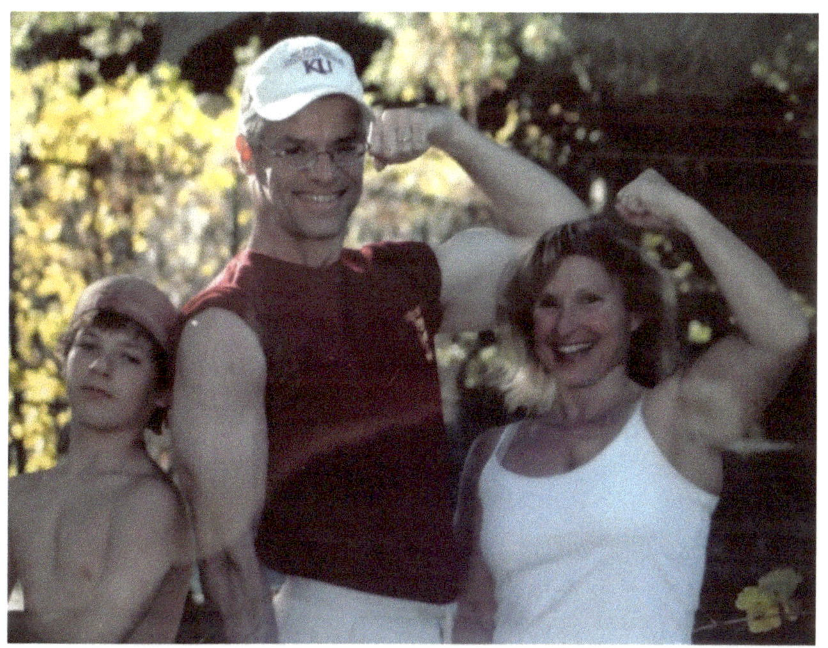

2008: Me (at age forty-seven) with my
wife, Diane, and son, Brandon

CHAPTER 6

The Fifties

One of the challenges of getting older is all the aches and pains that show up, sometimes for no apparent reason. It's one thing when you injure yourself working out. But it's quite another when something starts hurting, and you have no idea why—very frustrating and annoying. But it happens, and when it does, you just have to deal with it as best you can.

For me, one of the banes of my existence has been lower back pain. It plagued me for years and occasionally still does. Sometimes, I would tweak it when working out. Sometimes slouching in a chair would set it off. So I learned to be vigilant, and now I always sit up straight. Other times, it would flare up at the most unexpected times. For example, on several occasions, it tightened up on me when I was just standing around doing nothing. Not cool.

I had pretty much resigned myself to the fact that frequent lower back pain was, unfortunately, going to be with me for the rest of my life, but then, a miracle happened.

While skimming through a book on back pain one day, I learned that much, if not most, lower back pain is caused by differential tightening of the hamstrings. The book also included a stretch for the hamstrings, which I started doing several times a day. Within a week, the lower back pain was gone! I went from having some level of back pain most of the time to being pain-free most of the time. Behold, the miracle! I continue to do the stretch twice daily in maintenance mode. More frequently when my back infrequently acts up. Also I've shared it with others every chance I get, and I've helped them with their lower back pain, too! So sometimes the solution may be out there, but it just takes some time to find it.

In my fifties, along with the aches and pains, I also noticed that my stamina wasn't as good as it once was. So I made some more adjustments to my routine. In the past, I would typically lift weights and do cardio all in the same workout. But now, I typically didn't feel like I had enough stamina to hit both effectively, so I broke it up. I started alternating weight days and cardio days, which definitely helped. Again, the importance of listening to your body and adjusting your routine accordingly.

The two biggest workout challenges I would confront arrived while I was in my fifties. The first of these challenges was when my wonderful wife developed early-onset Alzheimer's. Throughout most of my fifties, it wasn't a big deal. She was increasingly forgetful, but our life together was still pretty good. She was forced to stop working on September 23, 2014. I'll never forget that day. For the next five years, she was still doing well enough that I could leave her alone for sixty to ninety minutes to go to the gym and work out, but things would get worse; more on that later.

Then, when I was fifty-nine, the other big challenge arrived in March of 2020. That was the COVID-19 pandemic. The first several months of the pandemic were a scary time. And for me, being a bit of a germaphobe, it was particularly scary. Not only was I afraid of getting COVID-19, but I was also worried about the implications. Would I get a bad case and require hospitalization? Would I get long Covid? If I did get sick, how would I be able to take care of my wife with Alzheimer's? A very scary time.

When the pandemic hit, and it became obvious it wasn't going to end any time soon, I cancelled my gym membership. I just didn't feel it was safe. So for the foreseeable future, I was going to work out at home.

Fortunately, I had created a bit of a home gym to help me get by if needed. My original thinking was to have enough equipment to allow me to get in a workout if the weather was bad or if work or family responsibilities prevented me from getting to the gym. I never thought it would be my everyday gym for almost three years. My home gym consisted of a set of dumbbells, an easy-curl bar, some plates for the bar, an adjustable bench, a stretchy band, and a cardio machine that simulated cross-country skiing. Then, with the first stimulus check we received early in the pandemic, I bought a new stationary bike, and that's it. That was all I had to work with. So to get effective workouts, I had to get really creative. For example, to do effective, full-range rows on a back day, I elevated the bench on cement blocks and duct-taped extra plates to the dumbbells. Whatever it takes to get a good workout! During the pandemic, my home gym was my salvation.

Remember this: Do what you can when you can. When it comes to your health, doing something is always better than doing nothing.

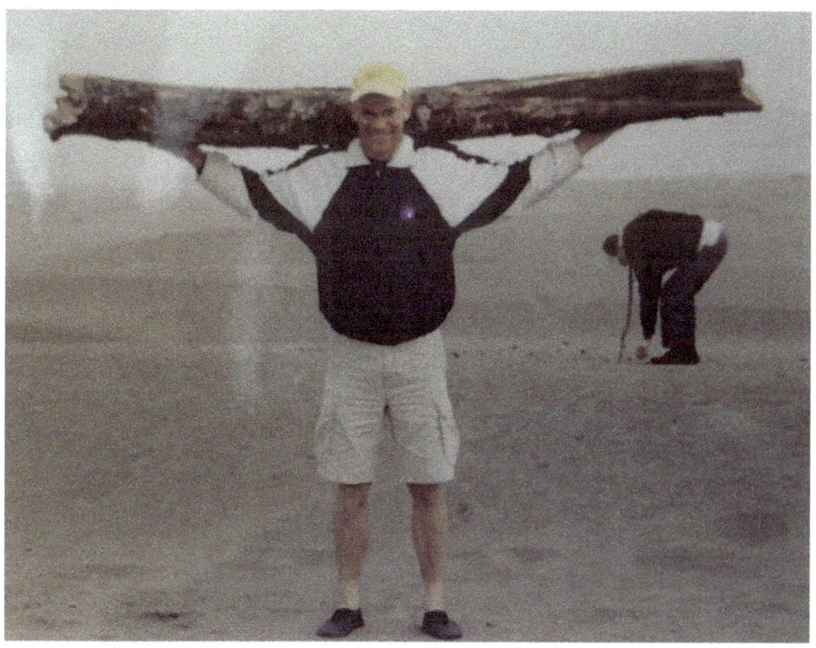

2011: I performed a feat of strength at age fifty.

CHAPTER 7

The Sixties

As I started my sixties, my life was not great. My wife's condition was continuing to deteriorate. Our relationship had now degraded from what once was an idyllic husband and wife partnership to what now could best be described as a strained parent-child relationship. We no longer had meaningful conversations, and she was increasingly incapable of doing even simple household tasks. I was no longer able to work full-time because of the increasing demands her care placed on me. I did, however, continue to work part-time from home.

I cared for my wife at home as long as I could. Maybe longer than I should have. During the last few months of her time at home, it was getting harder to work out. I was trying to work out and watch her at the same time. Eventually, I had to resort to locking us in the bedroom where my home gym is located. She liked coloring, so I would set her up with her coloring book and pencils. That would often, but not always, occupy her so I could do my workout. This was the most challenging time of my life, but I never missed a workout! I placed my wife in a care facility on May 23, 2022. Another day I will never forget. I cried that day.

Meanwhile, the COVID-19 pandemic continued to rage on. Despite my best efforts—five vaccine doses, wearing a mask everywhere, cancelled vacations, avoiding large indoor crowd situations—somehow, COVID-19 still got me in December 2022. It wasn't fun, but I survived it. In my case, I had a couple of bad days followed by shortness of breath for a good month. The upside was that now my immunity should be really good, at least for a few months.

After nearly three years of trying to avoid COVID-19, and after having COVID-19, I decided it was finally time to get back out there and rejoin the gym. It was great to be back. It was fun to reconnect with all my gym friends. And it was great to finally have variety in my workouts again, which definitely provided a boost to my motivation.

And now, a public service announcement: one of my pet peeves at the gym is people who don't put their weights back. They don't unload weight machines. They don't put their dumbbells back in the right place on the rack, or worse, they leave their dumbbells lying around on the floor. In addition to being inconsiderate, that's also a tripping hazard (which I can tell you from personal experience)—come on, people! Practice good gym etiquette. No excuses!

On a lighter note, I want to comment on all the different types of gym clientele that I've encountered over the years—quite the assortment.

I'm probably missing something, but here's what came to mind in no particular order:

1. Meatheads: These specimens only care about using as much weight as possible, technique be damned.
2. Young guns: Depending on their age, they may or may not be well muscled, but typically, they are motivated and work hard.
3. Strutters: By their actions and (or) their attire, they strut their stuff and want people to notice them.
4. Socializers: For them, the workout is strictly optional.
5. Lifters without a clue: For these people, there is seemingly no rhyme or reason to what they do. They just flit around doing a set of this and a set of that. I doubt they ever get a real pump.
6. Campers: These are the equipment hogs.
7. Regular Joes: Regular people doing regular workouts.
8. Innovators: These are the ones who always seem to be doing unique and interesting exercises and routines.
9. Oldsters: God bless 'em. They show up and do what they can.
10. Bodybuilders: No explanation required. As the saying goes, it takes all kinds. For the record, I would categorize myself as a regular Joe, a motivated and hard-working regular Joe.

In my sixties, I also added walks to my list of physical activities. Partly, it was for the extra exercise. But it was also to just get out of the house and get some fresh air. There's a nice park just a block from my house, so I usually walk there.

In 2023, I discovered the wonderful world of pickleball! For those of you not familiar with it, pickleball is sort of a smaller version of tennis that's played on a smaller court, with a paddle instead of a racquet, a different ball, and different rules. Oftentimes, tennis courts are also now lined so you can play pickleball on the same court. I really like it. It's a fun way to get some exercise, socialize, and make some new friends—all good things. I highly recommend it!

As of 2023, I've been living a healthy and active lifestyle for forty-five years. I'm determined to continue living a healthy and active lifestyle as long as I'm physically able to do so.

Remember this: It's never too late to start living a healthy and active lifestyle.

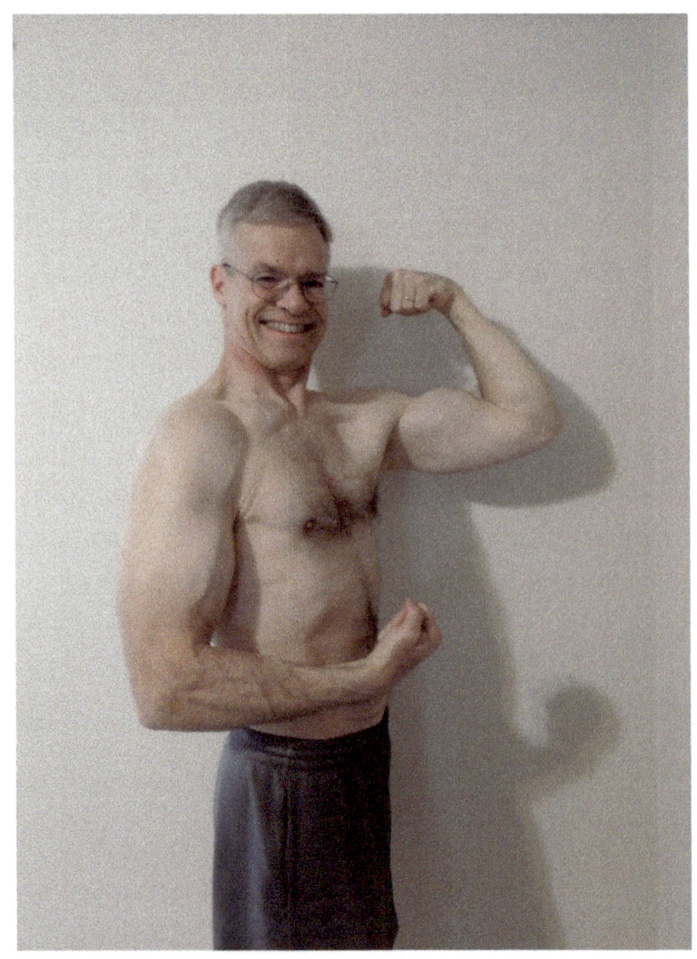

2021: Me on my sixtieth birthday

CHAPTER 8

Concluding Thoughts

I've had a wonderful and full life with many blessings and also some challenges. I give thanks every single day. I don't know how much time I have left. No one does. It may sound cliché, but the key is to make the most of each day. There are no do-overs. By living a healthy and active lifestyle, you will not only be able to make more of each day. You'll also likely get more days to enjoy. Life is so precious. Don't waste a single day of it. Get out there, make healthy and active choices, and live it!

ABOUT THE AUTHOR

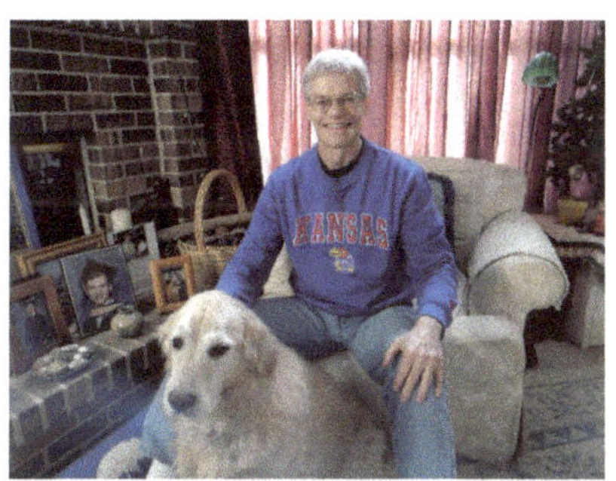

D r. Juracek was born in Lincoln and grew up in Omaha, Nebraska. In 1986, he moved to Lawrence, Kansas, to pursue his doctorate degree from the University of Kansas. After graduate school he stayed in Lawrence (where he still lives today) and worked as a research hydrologist for the U.S. Geological Survey (USGS). During his full-time career with USGS he authored or coauthored about 90 scientific publications on various topics including river science, reservoir science, and the effects of human activities on the environment. Currently, he works part time for USGS as he pursues nonscientific writing projects. He has one adult son and a golden retriever named Bo. Throughout his life he has always lived a healthy and active lifestyle. He believes in teaching by example and he's happy to report that his son has also adopted a healthy and active lifestyle. His motto is "the best way to get in shape is to never get out of shape." And that is how he has lived his life.